The Vibrant Keto Diet Meals Collection

Low Carb and Healthy Recipes To Boost Your Metabolism

Otis Fisher

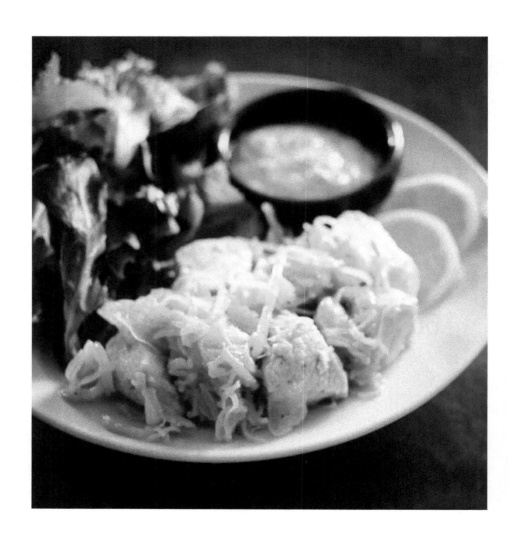

3

Readers acknowledge that the author is not engaging in the rendering of legal, financial, medical or professional advice. The content within this book has been derived from various sources. Please consult a licensed professional before attempting any techniques outlined in this book.

By reading this document, the reader agrees that under no circumstances is the author responsible for any losses, direct or indirect, which are incurred as a result of the use of information contained within this document, including, but not limited to, — errors, omissions, or inaccuracies.

Table of contents

Zucchini and Onion Chaffles

Preparation Time: 5 minutes

Cooking Time: 16 minutes

Servings: 4

Ingredients

- 2 cups zucchini, grated and squeezed
- 1/2 cup onion, grated and squeezed
- 2 organic eggs
- 1/2 cup Mozzarella cheese, shredded
- 1/2 cup Parmesan cheese, grated

Directions:

1. Preheat a Chaffle iron and then grease it.
2. In a medium bowl, set all ingredients and, mix until well combined.
3. Place 1/4 of the mixture into preheated Chaffle iron and Cooking for about 4 minutes or until golden brown.
4. Repeat with the remaining mixture.
5. Serve warm.

Nutrition:

Calories: 92

Net Carb: 2.

Fat: 5.3g

Saturated Fat: 2.3g

Carbohydrates: 3.5g

Dietary Fiber: 0.9g

Sugar: 1.8g

Protein: 8.6g

Jalapeño Chaffles

Preparation Time: 5 minutes

Cooking Time: 10 minutes

Servings: 2

Ingredients

- 1 organic egg, beaten
- 1/2 cup Cheddar cheese, shredded
- 1/2 tablespoon jalapeño pepper, chopped
- Salt, to taste

Directions:

1. Preheat a mini Chaffle iron and then grease it.
2. In a medium bowl, set all ingredients and with a fork, mix until well combined.
3. Set half of the mixture into preheated Chaffle iron and Cooking for about 5 minutes or until golden brown.
4. Repeat with the remaining mixture.
5. Serve warm.

Nutrition

Calories: 14et

Carb: 0.6g

Fat: 11.6g

Saturated Fat: 6.6g

Carbohydrates: 0.6g

Dietary Fiber: 0g

Sugar: 0.4g

Protein: 9.8g

Three-cheeses Herbed Chaffles

Preparation Time: 5 minutes

Cooking Time: 12 minutes

Servings: 4

Ingredients

- 4 tablespoons almond flour
- 1 tablespoon coconut flour
- 1 teaspoon mixed dried herbs
- 1/2 teaspoon organic baking powder
- 1/4 teaspoon garlic powder
- 1/4 teaspoon onion powder
- Salt and freshly ground black pepper
- 1/4 cup cream cheese, softened
- 3 large organic eggs
- 1/2 cup Cheddar cheese, grated
- 1/3 cup Parmesan cheese, grated

Directions:

1. Preheat a Chaffle iron and then grease it.
2. In a bowl, mix together the flours, dried herbs, baking powder and seasoning and mix well.
3. In a separate bowl, merge cream cheese and eggs and beat until well combined.
4. Add the flour mixture, cheddar and Parmesan cheese and mix until well combined.

5. Place the desired amount of the mixture into preheated Chaffle iron and Cooking for about 2-3 minutes or until golden brown.
6. Repeat with the remaining mixture.
7. Serve warm.

Nutrition:

Calories: 240

Net Carb: 2.6g

Fat: 19gSaturated

Fat: 5g

Carbohydrates: 4g

Dietary Fiber: 1.6g

Sugar: 0.7g

Protein: 12.3g

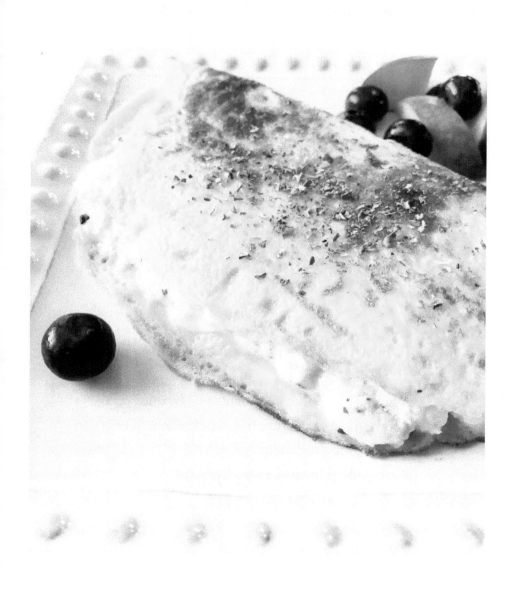

Pumpkin Chaffles with Choco Chips

Preparation time: 6 minutes

Cooking Time: 12 Minutes

Servings: 2

Ingredients:

- 1 egg
- 1/2 cup shredded mozzarella cheese
- 4 teaspoons pureed pumpkin
- 1/4 teaspoon pumpkin pie spice
- 2 tablespoons sweetener
- 1 tablespoon almond flour
- 4 teaspoons chocolate chips (sugar-free)

Directions:

1. Turn your Chaffle maker on.
2. In a bowl, set the egg and stir in the pureed pumpkin.
3. Mix well.
4. Add the rest of the ingredients one by one.
5. Pour 1/3 of the mixture to your Chaffle maker.
6. Cooking for 4 minutes.
7. Repeat the same steps with the remaining mixture.

Nutrition

Calories 93

Total Fat 7 g

Saturated Fat 3 g

Cholesterol 69 mg

Sodium 13mg

Potassium 48 mg

Total Carbohydrate 2 g

Dietary Fiber 1 g

Protein 7 g Total

Sugars 1 g

Pumpkin Cheesecake Chaffle

Preparation time: 10 minutes

Cooking Time: 15 Minutes

Servings: 2

Ingredients:

For chaffle:

- 1 egg
- 1/2 tsp. vanilla
- 1/2 tsp. baking powder, gluten-free
- 1/4 tsp. pumpkin spice
- 1 tsp. cream cheese, softened
- 2 tsp. heavy cream
- 1 tbsp. Swerve
- 1 tbsp. almond flour
- 2 tsp. pumpkin puree
- 1/2 cup mozzarella cheese, shredded

For filling:

- 1/4 tsp. vanilla
- 1 tbsp. Swerve
- 2 tbsp. cream cheese

Directions:

1. Preheat your mini Chaffle maker.
2. In a small bowl, mix all chaffle ingredients.
3. Spray Chaffle maker with Cooking spray.

4. Pour half batter in the hot Chaffle maker and Cooking for 3-5 minutes. Repeat with the remaining batter.
5. In a small bowl, combine all filling ingredients.
6. Spread filling mixture between two chaffles and place in the fridge for 10 minutes.
7. Serve and enjoy.

Nutrition

Calories 107

Fat 7.2

Carbohydrates 5

Sugar 0.7

Protein 6.7

Cholesterol 93 Mg

Quick and Easy Blueberry Chaffle

Preparation time: 10 minutes

Cooking Time: 15 Minutes

Servings: 2

Ingredients:

- 1 egg, lightly beaten
- 1/4 cup blueberries
- 1/2 tsp. vanilla
- 1 oz. cream cheese
- 1/4 tsp. baking powder, gluten-free
- 4 tsp. Swerve
- 1 tbsp. coconut flour

Directions:

1. Preheat your Chaffle maker.
2. In a small bowl, merge coconut flour, baking powder, and Swerve until well combined.
3. Add vanilla, cream cheese, egg, and vanilla and whisk until combined.
4. Spray Chaffle maker with Cooking spray.
5. Pour half batter in the hot Chaffle maker and top with 4- blueberries and Cooking for 4-5 minutes until golden brown. Repeat with the remaining batter.
6. Serve and enjoy.

Nutrition

Calories 135

Fat 8.2

Carbohydrates 11

Sugar 2.6

Protein 5

Cholesterol 9mg

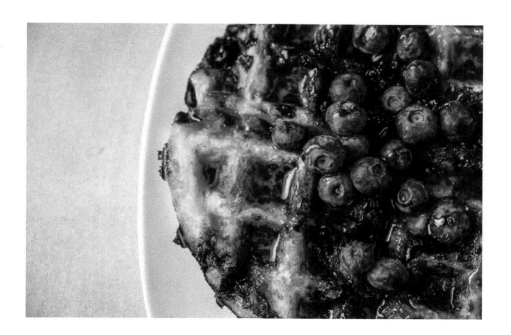

Raspberry and Chocolate Chaffle

Preparation time: 5 minutes

Cooking Time: 7-9 Minutes

Servings: 2

Ingredients:

Batter

- 4 eggs
- 2 ounces cream cheese, softened
- 2 ounces sour cream
- 1 teaspoon vanilla extract
- 5 tablespoons almond flour
- 1/4 cup cocoa powder
- 11/2 teaspoons baking powder
- 2 ounces fresh or frozen raspberries

Other

- 2 tablespoons butter to brush the Chaffle maker
- Fresh sprigs of mint to garnish

Directions:

1. Preheat the Chaffle maker.
2. Add the eggs, cream cheese and sour cream to a bowl and stir with a wire whisk until just combined.
3. Add the vanilla extract and mix until combined.
4. Stir in the almond flour, cocoa powder, and baking powder and mix until combined.

5. Add the raspberries and stir until combined.
6. Brush the heated Chaffle maker with butter and add a few tablespoons of the batter.
7. Close the lid and Cooking for about 8 minutes depending on your Chaffle maker.
8. Serve with fresh sprigs of mint.

Nutrition

Calories 270

Fat 23 G

Carbs 8.G

Sugar 1.3 G

Protein 10.2 G

Sodium 158 Mg

Red Velvet Chaffle

Preparation time: 6 minutes

Cooking Time: 12 Minutes

Servings: 2

Ingredients:

- 1 egg
- 1/4 cup mozzarella cheese, shredded
- 1 oz. cream cheese
- 4 tablespoons almond flour
- 1 teaspoon baking powder
- 2 teaspoons sweetener
- 1 teaspoon red velvet extract
- 2 tablespoons cocoa powder

Directions:

1. Combine all the ingredients in a bowl.
2. Plug in your Chaffle maker.
3. Set some of the batter into the Chaffle maker.
4. Seal and Cooking for minutes.
5. Open and transfer to a plate.
6. Repeat the steps with the remaining batter.

Nutrition

Calories 126

Total Fat 10.1g

Saturated Fat 3.4g

Cholesterol 66mg

Sodium 68mg

Potassium 290mg

Total Carbohydrate 6.5g

Dietary Fiber 2.8g

Protein 5.9g

Total Sugars 0.2g

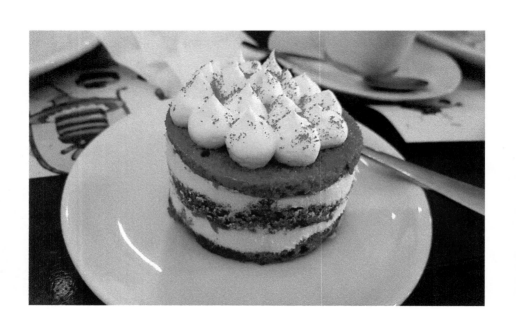

Sausage and Egg Chaffle Sandwich

Preparation time: 10 minutes

Cooking Time: 10 Minutes

Servings: 2

Ingredients:

- 2 basics Cooked chaffles
- 1 tablespoon olive oil
- 1 sausage, sliced into rounds
- 1 egg

Directions:

1. Set olive oil into your pan over medium heat.
2. Put it over medium heat.
3. Add the sausage and Cooking until brown on both sides.
4. Put the sausage rounds on top of one chaffle.
5. Cooking the egg in the same pan without mixing.
6. Place on top of the sausage rounds.
7. Top with another chaffle.

Nutrition

Calories 332

Total Fat 21.6g

Saturated Fat 4.4g

Cholesterol 139mg

Potassium 16g

Sodium 463mg

Total Carbohydrate 24.9g

Dietary Fiber 0g

Protein 10g

Total Sugars 0.2g

Sausage and Pepperoni Chaffle Sandwich

Preparation time: 8 minutes

Cooking Time: 10 Minutes

Servings: 2

Ingredients:

Cooking spray

- 2 cereal sausage, sliced into rounds
- 12 pieces pepperoni
- 6 mushroom slices
- 4 teaspoons mayonnaise
- 4 big white onion rings
- 4 basic chaffles

Directions:

1. Spray your skillet with oil.
2. Place over medium heat.
3. Cooking the sausage until brown on both sides.
4. Transfer on a plate.
5. Cooking the pepperoni and mushrooms for 2 minutes.
6. Spread mayo on top of the chaffle.
7. Top with the sausage, pepperoni mushrooms and onion rings.
8. Top with another chaffle.

Nutrition

Calories 373

Total Fat 24.4g

Saturated Fat 6g

Cholesterol 27mg

Sodium 717mg

Potassium 105mg

Total Carbohydrate 28g

Dietary Fiber 1.1g

Protein 8.1g

Total Sugars 4.5g

Simple Peanut Butter Chaffle

Preparation time: 5 minutes

Cooking Time: 7-9 Minutes

Servings: 2

Ingredients:

Batter

- 4 eggs
- 2 ounces cream cheese, softened
- 1/4 cup creamy peanut butter
- 1 teaspoon vanilla extract
- 2 tablespoons stevia
- 5 tablespoons almond flour

Other

- 1 tablespoon coconut oil to brush the Chaffle maker

Directions:

1. Preheat the Chaffle maker.
2. Add the eggs, cream cheese, and peanut butter to a bowl and stir with a wire whisk until just combined.
3. Add the vanilla extract and stevia and mix until combined.
4. Stir in the almond flour and stir until combined.
5. Brush the heated Chaffle maker with coconut oil and add a few tablespoons of the batter.
6. Close the lid and Cooking for about 7–8 minutes depending on your Chaffle maker.

7. Serve and enjoy.

Nutrition

Calories 291

Fat 24.9 G

Carbs 5.9 G

Sugar 2 G,

Protein 12.5 g

Sodium 1 mg

Super Easy Chocolate Chaffles

Preparation time: 10 minutes

Cooking Time: 5 minutes

Servings: 2

Ingredients:

- 1/4 cup unsweetened chocolate chips
- 1 egg
- 2 tbsps. almond flour
- 1/2 cup mozzarella cheese
- 1 tbsp. Greek yogurts
- 1/2 tsp. baking powder
- 1 tsp. stevia

Directions:

1. Switch on your square chaffle maker.
2. Spray the Chaffle maker with Cooking spray.
3. Mix together all recipe ingredients in a mixing bowl.
4. Spoon batter in a greased Chaffle maker and make two chaffles.
5. Once chaffles are Cooked, remove from the maker.
6. Serve with coconut cream, shredded chocolate, and nuts on top.
7. Enjoy!

Nutrition

Protein: 35

Fat: 59

Carbohydrates: 6

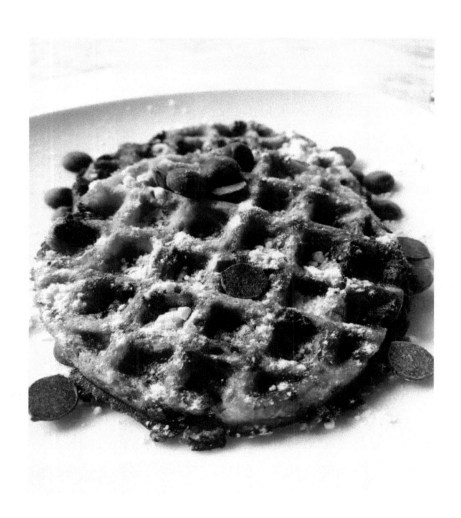

Sweet Vanilla Chocolate Chaffle

Preparation time: 10 minutes

Cooking Time: 10 Minutes

Servings: 2

Ingredients:

- 1 egg, lightly beaten
- 1/4 tsp. cinnamon
- 1/2 tsp. vanilla
- 1 tbsp. Swerve
- 2 tsp. unsweetened cocoa powder
- 1 tbsp. coconut flour
- 2 oz. cream cheese, softened

Directions:

1. Add all ingredients into the small bowl and mix until well combined.
2. Spray Chaffle maker with Cooking spray.
3. Pour batter in the hot Chaffle maker and Cooking until golden brown.
4. Serve and enjoy.

Nutrition

Calories 312

Fat 24

Carbohydrates 11.5

Sugar 0.8

Protein 11.6

Cholesterol 226 Mg

Keto Birthday Cake Chaffle with Sprinkles

Preparation Time: 10 minutes

Cooking Time: 7 minutes

Servings: 4

Ingredients

For chaffle cake:

- 2 eggs
- 1/4 almond flour
- 1 cup coconut powder
- 1 cup melted butter
- 2 tablespoons cream cheese
- 1 teaspoon cake butter extract
- 1 tsp. vanilla extract
- 2 tsp. baking powder
- 2 teaspoons confectionery sweetener or monk fruit
- 1/4 teaspoon xanthan powder whipped cream
- Vanilla frosting ingredients
- 1/2 cup heavy whipped cream
- 2 tablespoons sweetener or monk fruit
- 1/2 teaspoon vanilla extract

Direction

1. The mini Chaffle maker is preheated.

2. Add all the ingredients of the chaffle cake in a medium-sized blender and blend it to the top until it is smooth and creamy. Allow only a minute to sit with the batter. It may seem a little watery, but it's going to work well.

3. Add 2 to 3 tablespoons of batter to your Chaffle maker and Cooking until golden brown for about 2 to 3 minutes.

4. Start to frost the whipped vanilla cream in a separate bowl.

5. Add all the ingredients and mix with a hand mixer until thick and soft peaks are formed by the whipping cream.

6. Until frosting your cake, allow the keto birthday cake chaffles to cool completely. If you frost it too soon, the frosting will be melted.

Nutrition:

Calories 141

Fat 10.2g

Protein 4.7g

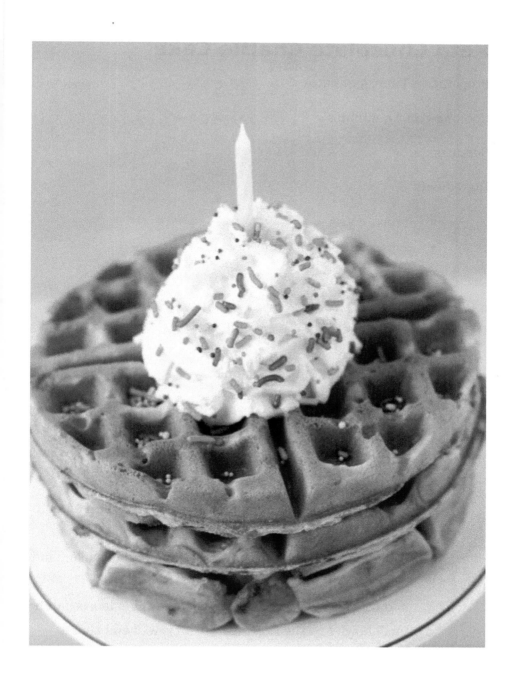

Keto Chocolate Chaffle Cake

Preparation Time: 5 minutes

Cooking Time: 5 minutes

Servings: 3

Ingredients

- 2 tbsp. cocoa
- 2 tbsp. monk fruit confectioner's
- 1 egg
- 1/4 teaspoon baking powder
- 1 tbsp. heavy whipped cream
- Frosted ingredients
- 2 tbsp. monk fruit confectioners
- 2 tbsp. cream cheese softens, room temperature
- 1/4 teaspoon transparent vanilla

Direction

1. Whip the egg.
2. Stir in rest of the ingredients then mix well until smooth and creamy.
3. Pour half of the batter into a mini Chaffle maker and Cooking until fully cooked for 2 1/2 to 3 minutes.
4. Add the sweetener, cream cheese, and vanilla in a separate small bowl. Mix the frosting until all is well embedded.
5. Lay out the frosting on the cake after it has cooled down to room temperature.

Nutrition:

Calories 120

Fat 10.5g

Protein 4.1g

Carrot Chaffle Cake

Preparation Time: 5 minutes

Cooking Time: 5 minutes

Servings: 6

Ingredients

- 1/2 cup chopped carrot
- 1 egg
- 2 t butter melted
- 2 t heavy whipped cream
- 3/4 cup almond flour
- 1 walnut chopped
- 2 t powder sweetener
- 2 tsp. cinnamon
- 1 tsp. pumpkin spice
- 1 tsp. baking powder
- Cream cheese frosting
- 4 oz. cream cheese softened
- 1/4 cup powdered sweetener
- 1 teaspoon of vanilla essence
- 1-2 t heavy whipped cream according to your preferred consistency

Directions

1. Mix dry ingredients such as almond flour, cinnamon, pumpkin spices, baking powder, powdered sweeteners, and walnut pieces.

2. Add the grated carrots, eggs, melted butter and cream.
3. Add a 3t batter to a preheated mini Chaffle maker. Cooking for 2 1 / 2-3 minutes.
4. Mix the frosted ingredients with a hand mixer with a whisk until well mixed
5. Stack Chaffles and add a frost between each layer!

Nutrition:

Calories 120

Fat 12g

Protein 5g

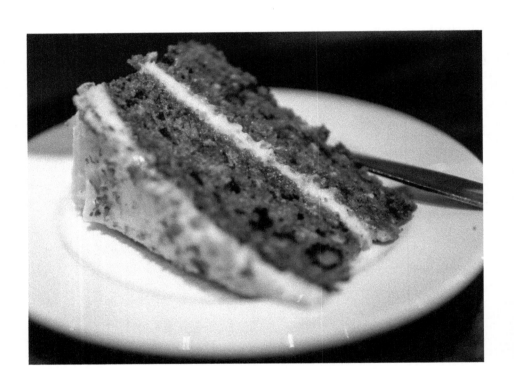

Easy Soft Cinnamon Rolls Chaffle Cake

Preparation Time: 5 minutes

Cooking Time: 12 minutes

Servings: 3

Ingredients

- 1 egg
- 1/2 cup mozzarella cheese
- 1/2 tsp. vanilla
- 1/2 tsp. cinnamon
- 1 tbsp. monk fruit confectioners blend

Directions

1. Put the eggs in a small bowl.
2. Add the remaining ingredients.
3. Spray to the Chaffle maker with a non-stick Cooking spray.
4. Make two chaffles.
5. Separate the mixture.
6. Cooking half of the mixture for about 4 minutes or until golden.
7. Notes added glaze: 1 tbsp. of cream cheese melted in a microwave for 15 seconds, and 1 tbsp. of monk fruit confectioner's mix. Mix it and spread it over the moist fabric.
8. Additional frosting: 1 tbsp. cream cheese (high temp), 1 tbsp. room temp butter (low temp) and 1 tbsp. monk fruit

confectioners' mix. Mix all the ingredients together and spread to the top of the cloth.

9. Top with optional frosting, glaze, nuts, sugar-free syrup, whipped cream or simply dust with monk fruit sweets.

Nutrition:

Calories 106

Fat 6.6g

Protein 8.2g

Banana Pudding Chaffle Cake

Preparation Time: 5 minutes

Cooking Time: 5 minutes

Servings: 2

Ingredients

- 1 large egg yolk
- 1/2 cup fresh cream
- 3 t powder sweetener
- 1 / 4-1 / 2 teaspoon xanthan gum
- 1/2 teaspoon banana extract
- Banana chaffle ingredients
- 1 oz. softened cream cheese
- 1/4 cup mozzarella cheese shredded
- 1 egg
- 1 teaspoon banana extract
- 2 t sweetener
- 1 tsp. baking powder
- 4 t almond flour

Direction

1. Mix heavy cream, powdered sweetener and egg yolk in a small pot. Whisk constantly until the sweetener has dissolved and the mixture is thick.
2. Cooking for 1 minute. Add xanthan gum and whisk.
3. Remove from heat, add a pinch of salt and banana extract and stir well.

4. Transfer to a glass dish and cover the pudding with plastic wrap. Refrigerate.
5. Mix all ingredients together. Cooking in a preheated mini Chaffle maker.

Nutrition:

Calories 130

Fat 13g

Protein 4g

Keto Peanut Butter Chaffle Cake

Preparation Time: 5 minutes

Cooking Time: 5 minutes

Servings: 2

Ingredients

for peanut butter chaffle:

- 2 tbs. sugar free peanut butter powder
- 2 tbs. monk fruit confectioner's
- 1 egg
- 1/4 teaspoon baking powder
- 1 tbs. heavy whipped cream
- 1/4 teaspoon peanut butter extract

Peanut butter frosting ingredients

- 2 tbs. monk fruit confectioners
- 1 tbs. butter softens, room temperature
- 1 tbs. unsweetened natural peanut butter or peanut butter powder
- •2 tbs. cream cheese softens, room temperature
- 1/4 tsp. vanilla

Directions

1. Serve the eggs.
2. Stir in remaining ingredients then mix well until smooth and creamy.

3. If you don't have peanut butter extract, you can skip it. It adds absolutely wonderful, more powerful peanut butter flavor and is worth investing in this extract.

4. Pour half of the butter into a mini Chaffle maker and Cooking for 2-3 minutes until it is completely Cooked.

5. In another small bowl, add sweetener, cream cheese, sugar-free natural peanut butter and vanilla. Mix frosting until everything is well incorporated.

6. When the Chaffle cake has completely cooled to room temperature, spread the frosting.

7. Or you can even pipe the frost!

8. Or you can warm up the frosting and pour 1/2 teaspoon of water to make the peanut butter pill and drizzle over the peanut butter chaffle! I like it anyway!

Nutrition:

Calories 92

Fat 7g

Protein 5.5g

Keto Italian Cream Chaffle Cake

Preparation Time: 5 minutes

Cooking Time: 3 minutes

Servings: 1

Ingredients

For sweet chaffle:

- 4 oz. cream cheese softens, room temperature
- 4 eggs
- 1 tablespoon butter
- 1 teaspoon of vanilla essence
- 1/2 teaspoon of cinnamon
- 1 tbsp. monk fruit sweetener or favorite keto approved sweetener
- 4 tablespoons coconut powder
- 1 tablespoon almond flour
- 1 1/2 cup baking powder
- 1 tablespoon coconut
- 1 walnut chopped

Italian cream frosting ingredients

- 2 oz. Cream cheese softens, room temperature
- 2 cups of butter room temp
- 2 tbs. monk fruit sweetener or favorite keto approved sweetener
- 1/2 teaspoon vanilla

Direction

1. Using medium blender, stir in cream cheese, eggs, melted butter, vanilla, sweeteners, coconut flour, almond flour, and baking powder. Optional: add shredded coconut and walnut to the mixture or save for matting. Both methods are great!
2. Incorporate the ingredients high until smooth and creamy.
3. Heat up mini Chaffle maker.
4. Pour in ingredients to the preheated Chaffle maker.
5. Cooking for 3 minutes until the Chaffle is complete.
6. Take out the chaffle and let cool.
7. Mix all the ingredients together and start frosting. Stir until smooth.
8. Once cooled, frost the cake.

Nutrition:

Calories 127

Fat 9.7g

Protein 5.3g

Keto Boston Cream Pie Chaffle Cake

Preparation Time: 10 minutes

Cooking Time: 5 minutes

Servings: 4

Ingredients

for chaffle cake:

2 eggs

- 1/4 cup almond flour
- Coconut flower 1 teaspoon
- 2 tablespoons of melted butter
- 2 tablespoons of cream cheese
- 20 drops of Boston cream extract
- 1/2 teaspoon of vanilla essence
- 1/2 teaspoon baking powder
- 2 tablespoons sweetener or monk fruit
- 1/4 teaspoon xanthan powder

Custard ingredients

- 1/2 cup fresh cream
- 1/2 teaspoon of vanilla essence
- 1/2 tbs. swerve confectioner's sweetener
- 2 yolks
- 1/8 teaspoon xanthan gum
- for ganache:
- 2 tbs. heavy whipped cream

- 2 tbs. unsweetened baking chocolate bar chopped
- 1 tbs. swerve confectioners' sweetener

Direction

1. Preheat the mini Chaffle iron to render the cake chops first.
2. Using a mixer, blend all the ingredients of the cake and blend until smooth. It's only supposed to take a few minutes.
3. Warm up heavy whipping cream to a boil on the stovetop. While it's dry, whisk the egg yolks together in a small separate dish.
4. Once the cream is boiling, add half of it to the egg yolks. Make sure you're whisking it together while you're slowly pouring it into the mixture.
5. Scourge egg and milk mixture to the rest of the cream in the stovetop pan and stir vigorously for 4 minutes.
6. Pull the custard off the heat and whisk in your vanilla and xanthan gum. Then set aside to cool and thicken.
7. Place the ganache ingredients in a small bowl. Microwave for about 20 seconds, stir. Repeat, if necessary. Careful not to overheat and roast the ganache. Just do it 20 seconds at a time until it's completely melted.
8. Assemble and enjoy your Boston cream pie chaffle cake!

Nutrition:

Calories 120

Fat 10.5g

Protein 3g

Keto Birthday Cake Chaffle

Preparation Time: 10 minutes

Cooking Time: 5 minutes

Servings: 4

Ingredients

for chaffle cake:

- 2 eggs
- 1/4 cup almond flour
- Coconut flower 1 teaspoon
- 2 tablespoons of melted butter
- 2 tablespoons of cream cheese
- 1 teaspoon cake batter extract
- 1/2 teaspoon of vanilla essence
- 1/2 teaspoon baking powder
- 2 tablespoons sweetener or monk fruit
- 1/4 teaspoon xanthan powder

Whipped cream vanilla frosting

- 1/2 cup fresh cream
- 2 tablespoons 2 tablespoons sweets sweetener or monk fruit
- 1/2 teaspoon of vanilla essence

Directions

1. Preheat mini Chaffle maker.

2. In a medium sized blender, add all the ingredients of the chaffle cake and blend high until smooth and creamy. Let the dough sit for only one minute. It may look a bit watery, but it works.

3. Add 2-3 tablespoons of dough to the Chaffle maker and Cooking for about 2-3 minutes until golden.

4. In another bowl, start making the whipped cream vanilla frosting.

5. Add all ingredients and mix with hand mixer until whipped cream thickens and soft peaks form.

6. Let the keto birthday cake chaffle cool completely before frosting the cake. If the frost is too early, the frost will melt.

Nutrition:

Calories 141

Fat 10.2g

Protein 4.7g

Keto Strawberry Shortcake Chaffle

Preparation Time: 2 minutes

Cooking Time: 4 minutes

Servings: 2

Ingredients

- 1 egg
- 1 tablespoon heavy whipped cream
- 1 tsp. coconut flour
- 2 tablespoons of Lecanto golden sweetener (use off wine)
- 1/2 teaspoon cake batter extract
- 1/4 teaspoon baking powder

Directions

1. Preheat the maker of mini Chaffles.
2. Combine all the ingredients of the chaffle in a small bowl.
3. Pour half of the mixture of the chaffle into the Chaffle iron center. Allow 3-5 minutes to Cooking. If the chaffle rises, lift the lid slightly for a couple of seconds until it begins to go back down and restore the lid as it finishes.
4. Carefully remove the second chaffle and repeat it. Let the chaffles sit for a couple of minutes to crisp up.
5. Add your desired and enjoyed amount of whipped cream and strawberries!

Nutrition:

Calories 268

Fat 11.8g

Protein 10g

Ham, Cheese and Tomato Chaffle Sandwich

Preparation Time: 5 minutes

Cooking Time: 10 minutes

Servings: 2

Ingredients:

- 1 teaspoon olive oil
- 2 slices ham
- 4 basic chaffles
- 1 tablespoon mayonnaise
- 2 slices Provolone cheese
- 1 tomato, sliced

Directions:

1. Pour in olive oil to a pan at medium heat.
2. Cooking the ham for 1 minute per side.
3. Spread the chaffles with mayonnaise.
4. Top with the ham, cheese and tomatoes.
5. Top with another chaffle to make a sandwich.

Nutrition:

Calories 198

Total Fat 14.7g

Protein 12.2g

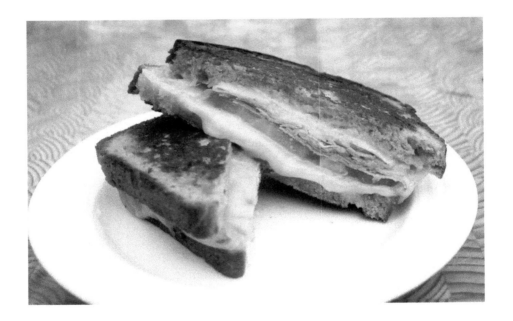

Chaffle with Sausage Gravy

Preparation Time: 5 minutes

Cooking Time: 15 minutes

Servings: 2

Ingredients:

- 1/4 cup sausage, Cooked
- 3 tablespoons chicken broth
- 2 teaspoons cream cheese
- 2 tablespoons heavy whipping cream
- 1/4 teaspoon garlic powder
- Pepper to taste
- 2 basic chaffles

Directions:

1. Add the sausage, broth, cream cheese, cream, garlic powder and pepper to a pan over medium heat.
2. Allow to boil then lower the heat.
3. Simmer for 10 minutes until thickened.
4. Pour the gravy on top of the basic chaffles
5. Serve.

Nutrition:

Calories 212

Total Fat 17g

Protein 11g

Barbecue Chaffle

Preparation Time: 5 minutes

Cooking Time: 8 minutes

Servings: 2

Ingredients:

- 1 egg, beaten
- 1/2 cup cheddar cheese, shredded
- 1/2 teaspoon barbecue sauce
- 1/4 teaspoon baking powder

Directions:

1. Plug in your Chaffle maker to preheat.
2. Mix all the ingredients in a bowl.
3. Pour half of the mixture to your Chaffle maker.
4. Cover and Cooking for 4 minutes.
5. Repeat the same steps for the next barbecue chaffle.

Nutrition:

Calories 295

Total Fat 23g

Protein 20g

Bacon and Chicken Ranch Chaffle

Preparation Time: 5 minutes

Cooking Time: 8 minutes

Servings: 2

Ingredients:

1 egg

- 1/4 cup chicken cubes, Cooked
- 1 slice bacon, Cooked and chopped
- 1/4 cup cheddar cheese, shredded
- 1 teaspoon ranch dressing powder

Directions:

1. Preheat your Chaffle maker.
2. In a bowl, mix all the ingredients.
3. Pour in half of the batter to your Chaffle maker.
4. Cover and Cooking for 4 minutes.
5. Make the second chaffle using the same steps.

Nutrition:

Calories 200

Total Fat 14 g

Protein 16 g

Cheeseburger Chaffle

Preparation Time: 15 minutes

Cooking Time: 15 minutes

Servings: 2

Ingredients:

- 1 lb. ground beef
- 1 onion, minced
- 1 tsp. parsley, chopped
- 1 egg, beaten
- Salt and pepper to taste
- 1 tablespoon olive oil
- 4 basic chaffles
- 2 lettuce leaves
- 2 cheese slices
- 1 tablespoon dill pickles
- Ketchup
- Mayonnaise

Directions:

1. Incorporate ground beef, onion, parsley, egg, salt and pepper.
2. Mix well.
3. Form 2 thick patties.
4. Add olive oil to the pan.
5. Place the pan over medium heat.

6. Cooking the patty for 3 to 5 minutes per side or until fully cooked.
7. Place the patty on top of each chaffle.
8. Top with lettuce, cheese and pickles.
9. Squirt ketchup and mayo over the patty and veggies.
10. Top with another chaffle.

Nutrition:

Calories 325

Total Fat 16.3g

Protein 39.6g

Savory Beef Chaffle

Preparation Time: 10 minutes

Cooking Time: 15 minutes

Servings: 2

Ingredients:

- 1 teaspoon olive oil
- 2 cups ground beef
- Garlic salt to taste
- 1 red bell pepper, sliced into strips
- 1 green bell pepper, sliced into strips
- 1 onion, minced
- 1 bay leaf
- 2 garlic chaffles
- Butter

Directions:

1. Put your pan over medium heat.
2. Add the olive oil and Cooking ground beef until brown.
3. Season with garlic salt and add bay leaf.
4. Drain the fat, transfer to a plate and set aside.
5. Discard the bay leaf.
6. In the same pan, Cooking the onion and bell peppers for 2 minutes.
7. Put the beef back to the pan.
8. Heat for 1 minute.
9. Spread butter on top of the chaffle.

10. Add the ground beef and veggies.

11. Roll or fold the chaffle.

Nutrition:

Calories 220 Total Fat 17.8g

Protein 27.1g

Bruschetta Chaffle

Preparation Time: 5 minutes

Cooking Time: 5 minutes

Servings: 2

Ingredients:

- 2 basic chaffles
- 2 tablespoons sugar-free marinara sauce
- 2 tablespoons mozzarella, shredded
- 1 tablespoon olives, sliced
- 1 tomato sliced
- 1 tablespoon keto friendly pesto sauce
- Basil leaves

Directions:

1. Spread marinara sauce on each chaffle.
2. Spoon pesto and spread on top of the marinara sauce.
3. Top with the tomato, olives and mozzarella.
4. Bake in the oven for 3 minutes or until the cheese has melted.
5. Garnish with basil.
6. Serve and enjoy.

Nutrition:

Calories 182

Total Fat 11g

Protein 16.8g

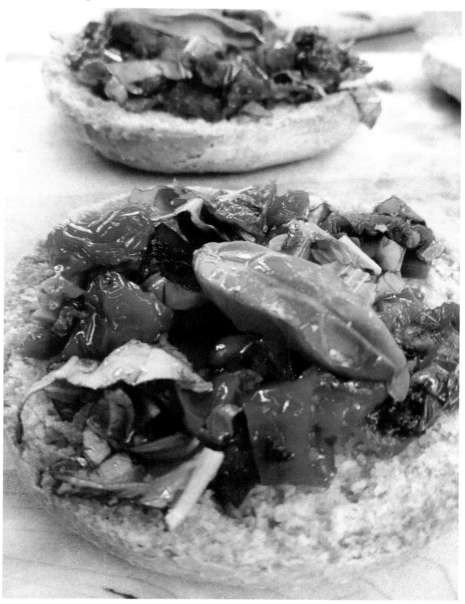

Hot Dog Chaffles

Preparation Time: 15 minutes

Cooking Time: 14 minutes

Servings: 2

Ingredients:

- 1 egg, beaten
- 1 cup finely grated cheddar cheese
- 2 hot dog sausages, cooked
- Mustard dressing for topping
- 8 pickle slices

Directions:

1. Preheat the Chaffle iron.
2. Scourge egg and cheddar cheese.
3. Open the iron and add half of the mixture. Close and Cooking until crispy, 7 minutes.
4. Transfer the chaffle to a plate and make a second chaffle in the same manner.
5. To serve, top each chaffle with a sausage, swirl the mustard dressing on top, and then divide the pickle slices on top.
6. Enjoy!

Nutrition:

Calories 231

Fats 18.29g

Protein 13.39g

Pulled Pork Chaffle

Preparation Time: 20 minutes

Cooking Time: 28 minutes

Servings: 4

Ingredients:

- 2 eggs, beaten
- 1 cup finely grated cheddar cheese
- 1/4 tsp. baking powder
- 2 cups Cooked and shredded pork
- 1 tbsp. sugar-free BBQ sauce
- 2 cups shredded coleslaw mix
- 2 tbsp. apple cider vinegar
- 1/2 tsp. salt
- 1/4 cup ranch dressing

Directions:

1. Preheat the Chaffle iron.
2. In a medium bowl, mix the eggs, cheddar cheese, and baking powder.
3. Open the iron and add a quarter of the mixture. Close and Cooking until crispy, 7 minutes.
4. Transfer the chaffle to a plate and make 3 more chaffles in the same manner.
5. Meanwhile, in another medium bowl, mix the pulled pork with the BBQ sauce until well combined. Set aside.

6. Also, mix the coleslaw mix, apple cider vinegar, salt, and ranch dressing in another medium bowl.

7. When the chaffles are ready, on two pieces, divide the pork and then top with the ranch coleslaw. Cover with the remaining chaffles and insert mini skewers to secure the sandwiches.

8. Enjoy.

Nutrition:

Calories 374

Fats 23.61g

Protein 28.05g

Ham and Cheddar Chaffles

Preparation Time: 15 minutes

Cooking Time: 28 minutes

Servings: 4

Ingredients:

- 1 cup finely shredded parsnips, steamed
- 8 oz. ham, diced
- 2 eggs, beaten
- 1 1/2 cups cheddar cheese
- 1/2 tsp. garlic powder
- 2 tbsp. chopped fresh parsley leaves
- 1/4 tsp. smoked paprika
- 1/2 tsp. dried thyme

Direction:

1. Preparation the Chaffle iron.
2. Incorporate all the ingredients.
3. Open the iron, lightly grease with Cooking spray and pour in a quarter of the mixture.
4. Close the iron and Cooking until crispy, 7 minutes.
5. Remove the chaffle onto a plate and set aside.
6. Make three more chaffles using the remaining mixture.
7. Serve.

Nutrition:

Calories 506

Fats 24.05g

Protein 42.74g

Turkey in Lemon Sauce Chaffle

Preparation Time: 5 minutes

Cooking Time: 18 minutes

Servings: 2

Ingredients

For chaffles:

- 1 large egg, beaten
- 1/2 cup cheddar cheese, shredded

For turkey:

- 1/2 cup of turkey breast, shredded
- 1/4 tsp. garlic powder
- 1/4 tsp. paprika powder
- 1 tsp. lemon juice
- A pinch of salt and black pepper
- 2 tbsp. heavy cream
- 1 tbsp. finely grated Parmesan cheese
- 1/2 tsp. fresh thyme, minced
- 1/2 tsp. fresh parsley, minced
- 1 tbsp. unsalted butter
- 1/2 cup chicken broth

Directions

For turkey:

1. In a saucepan over medium heat, Cooking the turkey breast in the unsalted butter part by part, for approx. 10 minutes. Season with a pinch of salt, black pepper and paprika.
2. Set aside the meat.
3. In the same saucepan, add garlic powder, chicken broth, heavy cream, parmesan cheese, lemon juice and thyme. Set to a boil and simmer until the sauce thickens. Add the turkey and mix well.

For chaffles:

1. Heat up the Chaffle maker.
2. Add all the chaffles ingredients to a small mixing bowl and stir until well combined.
3. Set half of the batter into the Chaffle maker and Cooking for 4 minutes until golden brown.
4. Top the chaffle with lemon sauce turkey.
5. Serve warm and enjoy!

Nutrition:

Calories: 264

Net Carb: 1.7g

Fat: 20g

Carbohydrates: 2.1g

Gourmet Grilled Prawns Chaffle

Preparation Time: 5 minutes

Cooking Time: 8 minutes

Servings: 2

Ingredients

For chaffles:

- 1 large egg, beaten
- 1/2 cup mozzarella cheese, shredded
- A pinch of salt

For topping:

- 6-8 grilled prawns
- 2 tsp. fresh parsley, minced
- 2 tbsp. butter, unsalted
- Lettuce leaves
- 1 small avocado, sliced
- 1 tomato, sliced

Directions:

1. Heat up the Chaffle maker.
2. Add all the chaffles ingredients to a small mixing bowl and stir until well combined.
3. Set half of the batter into the Chaffle maker and Cooking for 4 minutes until golden brown.

4. Spread the chaffles with butter. Top it with lettuce, tomato, slices of avocado and grilled prawns. Sprinkle with fresh parsley.

5. Serve immediately and enjoy!

Nutrition:

Calories: 145g

Net Carb: 0.5g

Fat: 11.6g

Carbohydrates: 0.5g

Dietary Fiber: 0g

Paprika and Scallion Chaffle

Preparation Time: 5 minutes

Cooking Time: 8 minutes

Servings: 2 chaffles

Ingredients

- 1 large egg, beaten
- 1/2 cup cheddar cheese, shredded
- 1/2 tbsp. paprika powder
- 1 tbsp. scallion, browned and thinly sliced

Directions:

1. Heat up the Chaffle maker.
2. Add all the chaffles ingredients to a small mixing bowl and stir until well combined.
3. Set half of the batter into the Chaffle maker and Cooking for 4 minutes, until brown.
4. Let cool for 3 minutes to let chaffles get crispy.
5. Serve and enjoy!

Nutrition

Calories: 119 kcal

Cholesterol: 111 mg

Carbohydrates: 2.7 g

Protein: 8.8 g

Anchovies Chaffle

Preparation Time: 5 minutes

Cooking Time: 8 minutes

Servings: 2

Ingredients:

- 1 large egg, beaten
- 1/2 cup shredded mozzarella cheese
- 4 filets anchovies, canned
- A pinch of black pepper

Directions:

1. Heat up the Chaffle maker.
2. Add all the chaffles ingredients to a small mixing bowl and stir until well combined.
3. Set half of the batter into the Chaffle maker and Cooking for 4 minutes until golden brown.
4. Serve and enjoy!

Nutrition:

Calories 235

Fats 20.62g

Carbs 5.9g

Net Carbs 5g

Keto Chaffle with Scallion Cream

Preparation Time: 5 minutes

Cooking Time: 8 minutes

Servings: 2

Ingredients

For chaffles:

- 1 large egg, beaten
- 1/2 cup of mozzarella cheese, shredded
- 2 tbsp. almond flour
- 1/4 tsp. baking powder

For scallion cream:

- 2 tbsp. cream cheese, softened
- 2 tbsp. scallion, browned and chopped

Directions:

1. In a small bowl, merge cream cheese and scallion until smooth. Set aside.
2. Heat up the mini Chaffle maker.
3. Add all the chaffles ingredients to a small mixing bowl and combine well.
4. Set half of the batter into the Chaffle maker and Cooking for 4 minutes until brown.
5. Let cool for 3 minutes to let chaffles get crispy.
6. Spread the chaffle with scallion cream.
7. Serve with cucumber pickles and enjoy!

Nutrition:

Calories: 77

Net Carb: 2.4g

Fat: 9.8g

Carbohydrates: 3.2g

Ground Pork Savory Chaffle

Preparation Time: 5 minutes

Cooking Time: 20 minutes

Servings: 2

Ingredients

For chaffles:

- 1 egg, beaten
- 1/2 cup shredded mozzarella cheese
- 1/2 tbsp. fresh basil, finely chopped
- A pinch of salt

For pork:

- 1 tsp. olive oil, extra virgin
- 2 cups ground pork
- 1 small red onion, chopped
- 1 tsp. fresh parsley, minced
- A pinch of salt and black pepper
- Ingredients for topping:
- 1 tbsp. keto mayonnaise
- 1 slice of cheddar cheese

Directions

For pork:

1. In a saucepan over low heat brown the onion in olive oil. Season with salt and pepper if needed. Add the ground pork

and the fresh parsley. Stir occasionally and Cooking until the meat is browned.

For chaffles:

1. Heat up the Chaffle maker.
2. Add egg, shredded cheddar cheese, a pinch of salt and basil in a small mixing bowl and combine well.
3. Set half of the batter into the Chaffle maker and Cooking for 4 minutes until brown.
4. Spread the chaffle with mayonnaise and garnish with ground pork. Add a slice of cheddar cheese.
5. Serve immediately and enjoy!

Nutrition

Calories: 417 kcal

Cholesterol: 170 mg

Carbohydrates: 13 g

Protein: 10 g

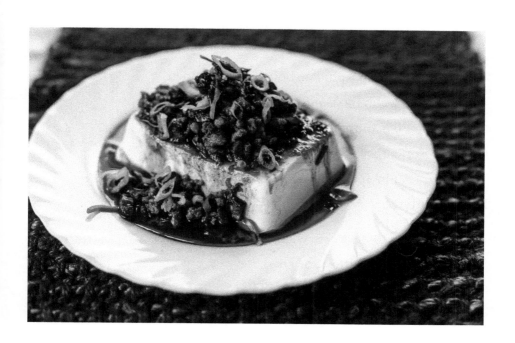

83

Dill Butter and Vegetables Chaffle

Preparation Time: 5 minutes

Cooking Time: 8 minutes

Servings: 2

Ingredients

For chaffles:

- 1 egg, beaten
- 1/2 tbsp. spinach, boiled and chopped
- 1/2 cup mozzarella cheese, shredded
- 1 tsp. onion, minced, browned
- 1/2 tbsp. broccoli, boiled and chopped
- A pinch of salt and pepper

For dill butter:

- 1/2 tbsp. cream cheese, softened
- 1 tbsp. butter, softened
- 1 tbsp. fresh dill, minced
- 1 tsp. lemon juice
- A pinch of salt and pepper

Directions

For dill butter:

1. Merge all the ingredients in a blender and whisk until creamy.

For chaffles:

1. Heat up the Chaffle maker.
2. Add all the chaffles ingredients to a small mixing bowl and stir until well combined.
3. Set half of the batter into the Chaffle maker and Cooking for 4 minutes until brown
4. Let cool for 3 minutes to let chaffles get crispy.
5. Serve with dill butter and enjoy!

Nutrition:

Calories: 145

Net Carb: 0.5g

Fat: 11.6g

Carbohydrates: 0.5g

Dietary Fiber: 0g

Blue Cheese Butter Chaffle

Preparation Time: 5 minutes

Cooking Time: 8 minutes

Servings: 2

Ingredients

For chaffles:

- 1 large egg, beaten
- 1/2 cup of mozzarella cheese, shredded
- 2 tbsp. almond flour
- 1/4 tsp. baking powder

For Blue cheese butter:

- 1 tbsp. butter, softened
- 2 tbsp. Blue cheese, shredded
- 1 tsp. fresh basil, chopped
- A pinch of salt and black pepper

Directions

For Blue cheese butter:

1. In a small mixing bowl, merge all the ingredients and stir well. Set aside.

For chaffles:

Heat up the Chaffle maker.

2. Add all the chaffles ingredients to a small mixing bowl and combine well.

3. Set half of the batter into the Chaffle maker and Cooking for 4 minutes until brown.
4. Let cool for 3 minutes to let chaffles get crispy.
5. Spread the chaffle with Blue cheese butter.
6. Serve and enjoy!

Nutrition:

Cal 215

Net Carbs 4g

Fat 15g

Protein 12g

Gourmet Chicken Salad Chaffle

Preparation Time: 5 minutes

Cooking Time: 8 minutes

Servings: 2

Ingredients

For chaffles:

- 1 large egg, beaten
- 1/2 cup shredded cheddar cheese

For chicken salad:

- 1/2 cup chicken, Cooking and shredded
- 1 tbsp. fresh celery, chopped
- 1 tsp. scallion, browned and minced
- 2 tbsp. avocado pulp, smashed
- 1 tsp. fresh basil, minced
- 2 tbsp. keto mayonnaise
- 1 tsp. keto mustard
- 1 tsp. lemon juice
- A pinch of salt and pepper

For filling:

- Spinach leaves
- 1 small hard-boiled egg, sliced
- 1 small tomato, sliced
- 1-2 pickled cucumbers, sliced

Directions

For chicken salad:

1. Merge all the ingredients in a mixing bowl and stir well. Set aside.

For chaffles:

1. Heat up the Chaffle maker.
2. Add egg and shredded cheese to a small mixing bowl and combine well.
3. Set half of the batter into the Chaffle maker and Cooking for 4 minutes until golden brown.
4. Garnish the chaffle with spinach leaves, chicken salad and 1 or 2 slices of hard-boiled egg. Add tomato and cucumbers.
5. Serve and enjoy!

Nutrition:

Cal 209

Net Carbs 2.7g;

Fat 17g

Protein 8g

Corned Beef Chaffle

Preparation Time: 5 minutes

Cooking Time: 8 minutes

Servings: 2

Ingredients

For chaffles:

- 1 large egg, beaten
- 1/2 cup of cheddar cheese, shredded
- 1 tbsp. almond flour
- 1/4 tsp. baking powder

For topping:

- 2 slices of corned beef
- 2 tbsp. keto mayonnaise
- A pinch of salt and black pepper

Directions:

1. Heat up the Chaffle maker.
2. Add all the chaffles ingredients to a small mixing bowl and stir until well combined.
3. Set half of the batter into the Chaffle maker and Cooking for 4 minutes until golden brown.
4. Let cool for 3 minutes to let chaffles get crispy.
5. Spread the chaffle with mayonnaise and top it with corned beef. Season with salt and pepper.
6. Serve and enjoy!

Nutrition

Calories: 261 kcal

Carbohydrates: 4 g net

Protein: 11.5 g

Fat: 22.2 g

Bacon and Jalapeño Chaffles

Preparation Time: 5 minutes

Cooking Time: 15 minutes

Servings: 5

Ingredients

- 3 tablespoons coconut flour
- 1 teaspoon organic baking powder
- 1/4 teaspoon salt
- 1/2 cup cream cheese, softened
- 3 large organic eggs
- 1 cup sharp Cheddar cheese, shredded
- 1 jalapeño pepper, seeded and chopped
- 3 Cooked bacon slices, crumbled

Directions:

1. Preheat a mini Chaffle iron and then grease it.
2. In a small bowl, set the flour, baking powder and salt and mix well.
3. In a large bowl, place the cream cheese and beat until light and fluffy.
4. Add the eggs and Cheddar cheese and beat until well combined.
5. Add the flour mixture and beat until combined.
6. Fold in the jalapeño pepper.
7. Divide the mixture into 5 portions.

8. Place 1 portion of the mixture into preheated Chaffle iron and Cooking for about 5 minutes or until golden brown.
9. Repeat with the remaining mixture.
10. Serve warm with the topping of bacon pieces.

Nutrition:

Calories: 249

Net Carb: 2.9g

Fat: 20.3gSaturated

Fat: 5g

Carbohydrates: 4.8g

Dietary Fiber: 1.9g

Sugar: 0.5g

Protein: 12.7g

Avocado Chaffle Toast

Preparation Time: 5 minutes

Cooking Time: 8 minutes

Servings: 2

Ingredients

- 1/2 avocado
- 1 egg
- 1/2 cup cheddar cheese, finely shredded
- 1 tbsp. almond flour
- 1 tsp. lemon juice, fresh
- Salt, ground pepper to taste
- Parmesan cheese, finely shredded for garnishing

Directions:

1. Warm up your mini Chaffle maker.
2. Mix the egg, almond flour with cheese in a small bowl.
3. For a crispy crust, add a teaspoon of shredded cheese to the Chaffle maker and Cooking for seconds.
4. Then, set the mixture into the Chaffle maker and Cooking for 5 minutes or until crispy.
5. Repeat with remaining batter.
6. Mash avocado with a fork until well combined and add lemon juice, salt, pepper
7. Top each chaffle with avocado mixture. Sprinkle with parmesan and enjoy!

Nutrition

Calories: 417 kcal

Cholesterol: 170 mg

Carbohydrates: 13 g

Protein: 10 g

Three-cheese Broccoli Chaffles

Preparation Time: 5 minutes

Cooking Time: 16 minutes

Servings: 4

Ingredients

- 1/2 cup Cooked broccoli, chopped finely
- 2 organic eggs, beaten
- 1/2 cup Cheddar cheese, shredded
- 1/2 cup Mozzarella cheese, shredded
- 2 tablespoons Parmesan cheese, grated
- 1/2 teaspoon onion powder

Directions:

1. Preheat a Chaffle iron and then grease it.
2. In a bowl, place all ingredients and mix until well merged.
3. Place half of the mixture into preheated Chaffle iron and Cooking for about 4 minutes or until golden brown.
4. Repeat with the remaining mixture.
5. Serve warm.

Nutrition:

Calories: 112

Net Carb: 1.2g

Fat: 8.1g

Saturated Fat: 4.3g

Carbohydrates: 1.5g

Dietary Fiber: 0.3g

Sugar: 0.5g

Protein: 8.

Bacon and Ham Chaffle Sandwich

Preparation Time: 5 minutes

Cooking Time: 5 minutes

Servings: 2

Ingredients

- 3 egg
- 1/2 cup grated Cheddar cheese
- 1 Tbsp. almond flour
- 1/2 tsp. baking powder
- For the toppings:
- 4 strips Cooked bacon
- 2 pieces Bibb lettuce
- 2 slices preferable ham
- 2 slices tomato

Directions:

1. Turn on Chaffle maker to heat and oil it with Cooking spray.
2. Combine all chaffle components in a small bowl.
3. Add around 1/4 of total batter to Chaffle maker and spread to fill the edges. Close and Cooking for 4 minutes.
4. Remove and let it cool on a rack.
5. Repeat for the second chaffle.
6. Top one chaffle with a tomato slice, a piece of lettuce, and bacon strips, and then cover it with second chaffle.
7. Plate and enjoy.

Nutrition:

Carbs: 5

Fat: 60 g

Protein: 31 g

Calories: 631

Burger Chaffle

Preparation Time: 5 minutes

Cooking Time: 10 minutes

Servings: 1

Ingredients

For the Cheeseburgers:

- 1/3 lb. beef, ground
- 1/2 tsp. garlic salt
- 3 slices American cheese

For the Chaffles:

- 1 large egg
- 1/2 cup mozzarella, finely shredded
- Salt and ground pepper to taste
- For the Big Mac Sauce:
- 2 tsp. mayonnaise
- 1 tsp. ketchup

To Assemble:

- 2 tbsp. lettuce, shredded
- 4 dill pickles
- 2 tsp. onion, minced

Directions:

1. Take your burger patties and place them on one chaffle. Top with shredded lettuce, onions and pickles.

2. Spread the sauce over the other chaffle and place it on top of the veggies, sauce side down.

3. Enjoy.

Nutrition:

Calories: 85

Fats: 56 g

Carbs: 8 g

Protein: 67 g

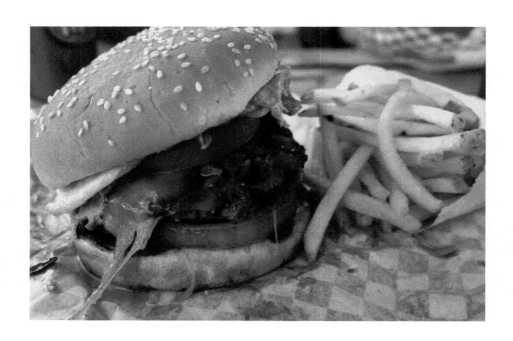

Bbq Chicken Chaffles

Preparation Time: 5 minutes

Cooking Time: 8 minutes

Servings: 2

Ingredients

- 1 1/3 cups grass-fed Cooked chicken, chopped
- 1/2 cup Cheddar cheese, shredded
- 1 tablespoon sugar-free BBQ sauce
- 1 organic egg, beaten
- 1 tablespoon almond flour

Directions:

1. Preheat a mini Chaffle iron and then grease it.
2. In a bowl, place all ingredients and mix until well merged.
3. Set half of the mixture into preheated Chaffle iron and Cooking for about 4 minutes or until golden brown.
4. Repeat with the remaining mixture.
5. Serve warm.

Nutrition:

Calories: 320

Net Carb: 3.

Fat: 16.3g

Saturated Fat: 7.6g

Carbohydrates: 4g

Dietary Fiber: 0.4g

Sugar: 2g

Protein: 36.9g

Avocado Chaffle

Preparation Time: 5 minutes

Cooking Time: 10 minutes

Servings: 2

Ingredients

- 1/2 avocado, sliced
- 1/2 tsp. lemon juice
- 1/8 tsp. salt
- 1/8 tsp. black pepper
- 1 egg
- 1/2 cup shredded cheese
- 1/4 crumbled feta cheese
- 1 cherry tomato, halved

Directions:

1. Merge together avocado, lemon juice, salt, and pepper until well-combined.
2. Turn on Chaffle maker to heat and oil it with Cooking spray.
3. Beat egg in a small mixing bowl.
4. Place 1/8 cup of cheese on Chaffle maker, then spread half of the egg mixture over it and top with 1/8 cup of cheese.
5. Close and Cooking for 3-4 minutes. Repeat for remaining batter.
6. Let chaffles cool for 3-4 minutes, and then spread avocado mix on top of each.
7. Top with crumbled feta and cherry tomato halves.

Nutrition

Carbs: 5 g

Fat: 19 g

Protein: 7 g

Calories: 232

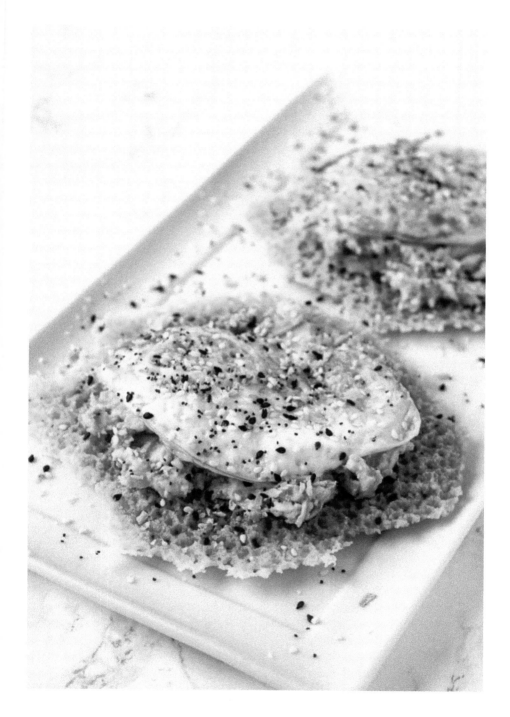

Lightning Source UK Ltd.
Milton Keynes UK
UKHW020812110621
385331UK00004B/93